THE BABYDUST METHOD

a guide to conceiving a girl or a boy

by Kathryn Taylor

Dedication

To my husband Joe, who is the love of my life and my biggest supporter. To my kids Jack and Emma, who are my sweet little angels and my inspiration for writing this book. To my mom Ellen, who helps me with absolutely everything.

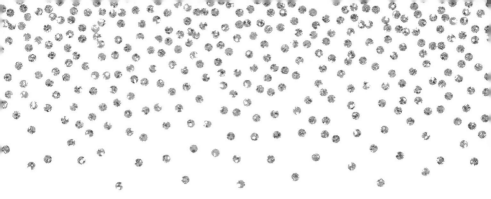

Contents

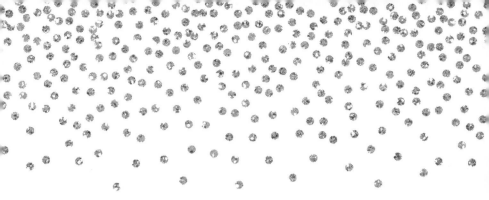

Foreword

Sex. I know, it's just as weird for me to type it as it is for you to read it. But, we're gonna talk about it — a lot. It's the topic of this whole book. No, I don't mean the actual sex you'll be having with your partner to conceive your baby. I mean "sex" as in girl or boy. And I don't mean "gender." Let's clear up the confusion right now. Sex refers to the physical characteristics and genetic makeup of a person, whereas gender refers to a person's behavior, social interaction with others, and role in society. Throughout this book, I will use the term sex instead of gender. The reason I'm making a hard distinction is because it is the crux of this book.

Before we begin to discuss sex-selection, I encourage you now to think about why you want a girl or a boy. Do you want to dress your daughter up in cute outfits and bows and play dolls with her? Do you want to watch football with your son and wrestle with him? I can't promise your child will do any of that. My daughter pulls the bows out of her hair one minute after I put them in. My son has no interest in even catching a ball, let alone sitting down to watch a football game. We're only talking about the sex here, not the gender. The sex of your baby only pertains to which sex organs your baby will have and how your baby will procreate one day.

In society, there is a strong preference for sex balancing, that is, maintaining a proper ratio of boys to girls in a family. It's no surprise that a mother of 5 girls would yearn for a little boy to add some masculinity to her brood. A father of all boys might want to have that special father-daughter relationship he's been missing. Researchers have theorized that the size of families might change if the sexes of their children had been controlled.[1] Many couples want to have at least one boy and at least one girl. Having more children than is desired, just to have one of each sex, puts a strain on families. Therefore, utilizing sex-selection methods can promote marital and familial harmony.

We all want to have control, especially when it comes to family. Creating a miniature version of yourself or your partner, I get it. I felt the same way when we began planning for our family. But once the baby gets here, you'll see. They will decide who they are, what toys they play with, what sports they are interested in (if any), the clothes they wear, the friends they have, and the choices they make. I can't help you with who they will turn out to be in life. That remains undetermined. Although I can't guarantee that you'll conceive the sex of your choice, what I *can* do is teach you how to dramatically increase your chances of conceiving a girl or a boy, by using *The Babydust Method.*

Several methods for influencing the sex of babies have been proposed over the years. I will explain those methods in detail, why each of them is flawed, why *The Babydust Method* is highly effective, and how you can use this completely natural method to more accurately choose the sex of your baby.

---

1   Ben-Porath, Y., and Welch, F. "Do sex preferences really matter?" *The Quarterly Journal of Economics* 90.2 (1976): 285.

Glossary of Terms

Throughout this book, and on the Facebook group, "The Babydust Method Group Forum," you will see several acronyms:

AF.......... Aunt Flo *(your period)*

BBT .... Basal Body Temperature

BD .... Bed Down or Baby Dance *(literally means having sex)*

BFN .... Big Fat Negative *(negative pregnancy test)*

BFP.......... Big Fat Positive *(positive pregnancy test!!!!)*

CD .... Cycle Day *(with day 1 being the first day of your period)*

CM .... Cervical Mucus

DD .... Dear Daughter *(your baby girl/female child)*

DF, DH, DP .. Dear Fiancé, Dear Husband, Dear Partner
(I'll be using DP throughout this book)

DPO......... Days Past Ovulation *(counting day 0 as the day of ovulation)*

DS........... Dear Son *(your baby boy/male child)*

DTD........ Doing the Dance/Deed *(also means having sex)*

DW.......... Dear Wife

FMU........ First Morning Urine

HCG........ Human Chorionic Gonadotropin *(pregnancy hormone)*

HPT .... Home Pregnancy Test

LH.......... Luteinizing Hormone *(ovulation hormone)*

O............ Ovulation

O'd .... Ovulated

OPK .... Ovulation Predictor Kit

POAS .... Pee On A Stick *(taking ovulation or pregnancy tests)*

TTC .... Trying To Conceive

2WW .... Two Week Wait *(the time between ovulation and your next period, when you're waiting to take a pregnancy test)*

And lastly, **"Babydust,"** which means sending good luck and best wishes to those trying to conceive a precious little baby :)

Babydust to all
XOXO,
Kathryn

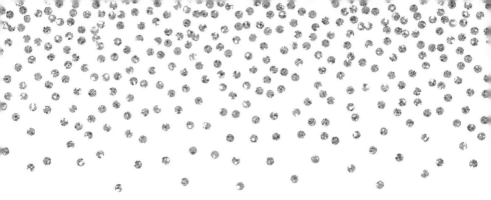

Getting Started

Mind

You're bringing another life, another soul into this world. Treat yourself right. Reduce stress, sleep better, focus on you, and envision your future baby and your future family. Focus your mind on what you want. Think about your gorgeous baby and all the fun things you'll do together. Get excited!

Get your relationships in order. Is there anything in your relationship with your partner that you need to work on? Any issues you need to talk through? Having a baby is one of the most challenging yet rewarding things you can do in life. Make sure you and your partner are ready to embark on this journey together.

Body

Your body is going to go through a ton of changes during the 9 months of pregnancy. You need to give it the fuel it needs to build your perfect little baby. You and your partner should aim to eliminate unnecessary prescription drugs (talk to your doctor first) as well as over-the-counter medicines such as, ibuprofen (Motrin, Advil), naproxen (Aleve), acetaminophen (Tylenol), and aspirin. DO take vitamins. A prenatal vitamin from the drug store will be just fine. It will contain the appropriate amounts of folic acid, vitamin D, calcium and B vitamins for pregnancy. Consider adding an iron supplement if your doctor agrees. In addition, omega-3 fatty acids like DHA are critical for your baby's brain development. Your body is going to be your baby's sole source of nutrients, so take care of yourself. Encourage your partner to take multivitamins as well.

Stop drinking alcohol, and quit smoking. We're all aware of the dangers associated with alcohol and smoking, especially while pregnant. Coffee consumption is up for debate. Most doctors recommend one cup of coffee or less per day. The problem here is that not all cups of coffee are created equal in terms of caffeine. It may be hard to open your eyes in the morning without that precious cup of coffee, especially with older kids running around, but my advice is to cut this one out. Sorry :)

You're going to gain weight. I know that doesn't sound like fun. Try to embrace it and remember that the extra weight is necessary to nourish your precious creation. It is a natural thing. Dieting or working out too hard can have a negative impact on your fertility and pregnancy.

If you're breastfeeding an older baby, you don't have to stop. That is something for you and your baby to decide. However, breastfeeding can alter your hormones, which could interfere with *The Babydust Method.* Also, it is a myth that if you're breastfeeding, you can't get pregnant, so please use condoms until you are ready to attempt sex-selection.

When to Start

You'll need to chart 3 consecutive menstrual cycles before you attempt sex-selection. Put on your lab coat and your scientist glasses, and get ready to record your cycle data in the back of this book, or on any blank calendar you'd prefer to use.

If you've had a baby within the last 6 months, or if you have just stopped breastfeeding, chart 3 extra cycles (6 cycles total) before you begin your sex-selection attempt. I know that sounds like a long time to wait before you try to conceive, but your hormones are going through intense changes during the months following birth and weaning, and this could throw off your timing.

With the exception of condoms, you must discontinue all other forms of birth control when you begin charting your cycles. No pills, no patches, no IUDs — just condoms. Your body needs time to get itself back to its normal state, so give yourself a month or two after you discontinue your birth control, before you start charting. Birth control prevents ovulation. *The Babydust Method* relies on tracking ovulation. It is absolutely essential that you are not on birth control during your charting cycles.

Are you ready? Excited? Nervous? Let's go over the existing sex-selection methods, what's wrong with them, and how *The Babydust Method* was born.

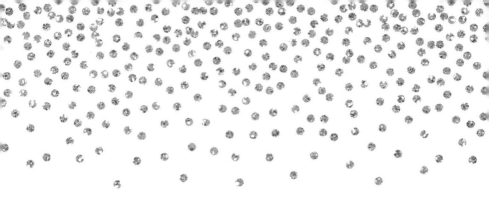

Other Sex-Selection Methods — Why They're Flawed

If you're like me, you've already googled, "How to conceive a girl or a boy," and gotten a headache reading all the diets, douches, and charts, including the Chinese Gender Chart — don't even get me started. It's a chart based on how old you are at the time of conception and what month you're conceiving in. It was found in an ancient Chinese tomb. Ya, it's wrong. Based on the chart, my boy would have been a girl and my girl would have been a boy. The sex-selection information online will make you go crazy. You'll buy lemon douches and meal plans, and end up frustrated and confused.

The Menstrual Cycle

Let's start by talking about your favorite friend — your period. The menstrual cycle is bounded by the first day of your period and the first day of your next period. The time in between these two dates is known as "your cycle." The average number of days in a cycle is

28. You may notice that the number of days in your cycle fluctuates by a day or two; one month it's 27 days, the next month it's 29 days, but it tends to hover around the same number. Or, you may notice you have irregular cycles, with one cycle lasting 24 days and the next cycle lasting 35 days.

The first half of your cycle is called the follicular phase. The first 1-5 days of this phase is called *menses*, aka bleeding. This is the time of the month where you are "on your period." Your uterus is shedding its lining and the estrogen in your body is slowly rising.

MENSTRUAL CYCLE

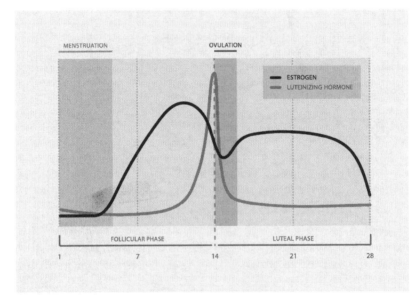

A peak in estrogen in the days leading up to the midpoint of your cycle results in the increase of another hormone called *luteinizing hormone*, aka LH. This usually occurs on day 14, but could occur between days 10 and 20, depending on the length of your cycle. LH is responsible for the release of the egg from your ovary, aka *ovulation*. After LH peaks, aka surges, ovulation will occur in approximately

24 hours. Most women ovulate between 12 and 48 hours after the LH surge, but 24 hours is the average.[2]

Ovulation marks the transition to the second half of your cycle, called the luteal phase. This phase starts with ovulation and ends with the start of your next period. Once the egg is released from your ovary, it travels down the fallopian tubes and waits for one lucky sperm to fertilize it. If the egg does not get fertilized within 12-24 hours, it will travel down into the uterus and will flow out through your vagina during your period. However, if the egg *does* get fertilized, this means the egg and sperm have fused together to become one cell, called a zygote. This is the moment of conception. From this point forward, that single fused cell will divide millions of times to become your baby.

The zygote quickly turns into a ball of cells called a blastocyst. After 6-12 days, the blastocyst implants itself into your uterine lining and begins to receive nutrients.[3] Even before you can take a pregnancy test, your baby is exposed to everything that is present in your blood, so it is extremely important that you have been diligently taking your vitamins and have discontinued using all dangerous or unnecessary substances.

The Science of Conception

The sex of the baby is determined at the moment of conception. A female baby has one X chromosome from her mom, and another X from her dad. A male baby has an X from his mom and a Y from his dad. Each egg in your body has one X chromosome. Sperm on the other hand, contain either an X chromosome, which would create a female baby, or a Y chromosome, which would create a male baby. It is the sperm alone that determines the sex of the baby.

---

2   "Ovulation kits & fertility monitors." *American Pregnancy Association.* N.p., 23 Apr. 2012. Web. 14 Mar. 2016.

3   "How soon after implantation do I get a positive pregnancy test?" *New Health Advisor,* N.p., n.d. Web. 14 Mar. 2016.

The Shettles Method —
What He Got Right, What He Got Wrong

In 1971, Dr. Landrum B. Shettles pioneered the idea of sex-selection. He observed sperm under a microscope and noted that some had small, pointed heads and others had large, rounded heads. He observed the smaller, pointier sperm swimming rapidly and theorized that these sperm contained a Y chromosome (male-producing sperm). He observed the larger, more rounded sperm swimming more slowly and theorized they had an X chromosome (female-producing sperm). He went on to postulate, that if the pointy-headed male sperm were so small and fast, they would reach the egg first, but they were probably weaker and would die quickly. The slower, hardier female sperm would take longer to reach the egg, but would survive longer than the male sperm would.

Dr. Shettles also theorized that acidity vs. alkalinity of the vaginal tract was important in sex-selection. Since he thought that the Y sperm were smaller and more fragile, he hypothesized that vaginal fluids that were acidic would kill the all the male sperm, leaving only the female sperm available to fertilize the egg. On the other hand, he theorized that vaginal fluids that were alkaline would allow both male and female sperm to survive, but only the faster swimming Y sperm would get to the egg first.

The secretions present at the entrance of the vagina are naturally more acidic than those found closest to the cervix. Therefore, Dr. Shettles postulated that certain sexual positions (such as entry from the rear, aka doggy-style) that fostered deeper penetration would deposit the sperm closer to the cervix, bypassing most of the acidic secretions in the vaginal tract, and favoring male sperm. Also, female orgasms tend to produce alkaline secretions, so having an orgasm before, during, or after the man's orgasm would favor boys as well. In order to conceive a girl, he thought couples should do the opposite, engaging in sexual positions (such as missionary) with shallow penetration, so the sperm would be deposited towards the acidic opening of the vagina. He also suggested that the female should avoid having an orgasm, in order to keep her vaginal secretions acidic.

Lastly, Dr. Shettles theorized that high sperm counts favor boys and low sperm counts favor girls. To conceive a boy, Dr. Shettles suggested abstaining from sex as long as possible in order to build up sperm count. Conversely, having sex frequently would reduce sperm count and result in a female baby. Specifically, to conceive a boy he recommended abstaining from sex during the first half of the menstrual cycle and then having sex one time on the day of ovulation. This would allow only the faster male sperm to reach the egg first, and would result in a male fetus. To conceive a girl, he recommended having sex frequently during the first half of the menstrual cycle until 2-3 days before ovulation and then stopping. This would allow enough time for all the male sperm to die off and would leave only the longer living female sperm waiting for the egg.[4]

Sounds plausible, right? The trouble is, in 1971 Dr. Shettles had no way of knowing which sperm contained an X and which contained a Y. The differences in X and Y sperm that Dr. Shettles observed under the microscope were actually *capacitated* and *uncapacitated* sperm.

What is capacitation, then? Fresh sperm are incapable of fertilizing an egg immediately. They must first undergo a series of physical changes to their outer membrane. These changes enable the sperm to fertilize the egg, increase sperm speed, and make the head of the sperm appear smaller and pointier under a microscope.[5] Dr. Shettles observed the smaller, pointier, supposed Y sperm moving more rapidly than the larger, rounder, supposed X sperm, because he was simply observing a batch of sperm that contained capacitated as well as uncapacitated sperm.

---

4   Shettles, L. B., and Rorvik, D. M. "How to choose the sex of your baby: the method best supported by scientific evidence." New York: Broadway, 2006.

5   Grant, V. J. "Entrenched misinformation about X and Y sperm." *BMJ* 332.7546 (2006): 916.

UNCAPACITATED VS. CAPACITATED SPERM

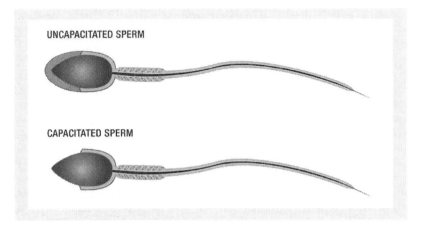

UNCAPACITATED SPERM

CAPACITATED SPERM

Scientists have continued to attempt to differentiate between X and Y sperm over the years, but contrary to Dr. Shettles' findings, studies have shown that there is no observable physical difference between X and Y sperm.[6] However, there is 2.8% less genetic material in the Y sperm, due to the smaller size of the Y chromosome,[7] but studies have shown that this small difference in the mass of the genetic material in the nucleus of the sperm cell does not result in any observable difference in sperm size.[8] Studies have also proven there is no relationship between acidity or alkalinity of the vaginal tract and the sex ratios of the resultant offspring.[9] Lastly, several studies have proven that X and Y sperm swim at the same speed,

6   Grant, V. J. "Entrenched misinformation about X and Y sperm." *BMJ* 332.7546 (2006): 916.

7   Johnson, L. A., Welch, G. R., Keyvanfar, K., Dorfmann, A., Fugger, E. F., and Schulman, J. D. "Gender preselection in humans? Flow cytometric separation of X and Y spermatozoa for the prevention of X-linked diseases." *Human Reproduction* 1993, 8: 1733-1739.

8   Hossain, A. M., Barik, S., and Kulkarni, P. M. "Lack of significant morphological differences between human X and Y spermatozoa and their precursor cells (spermatids) exposed to different prehybridization treatments." *Journal of Andrology* 2001; 22: 119-23.

9   Muehleis P.M. "The effects of altering the pH of seminal fluid on the sex ratio of rabbit off- spring." *Fertility and Sterility* 1976, 27: 1438-45.

which invalidates Dr. Shettles' original premise, upon which his entire sex selection method was based.[10][11]

Nevertheless, Dr. Shettles claims a 75% success rate using his girl method, and an 80% success rate using his boy method. The trouble is, these percentages were based primarily on parents who tried his method and then wrote letters to him or responded to his questionnaires. This data collection method created a huge selection bias. That is to say, his sample of women was not randomized and data was not collected in the controlled manner of a clinical trial, which is the method upon which the FDA, doctors, and the scientific community base their conclusions. The problem is, people who were excited that the method worked for them might have been more likely to write him a letter or respond to the questionnaire than the people for whom the method did not work, thus skewing his method's success rate in his favor.

Is Dr. Shettles wrong? Yes and no. Y sperm are not faster than X sperm, and Y sperm are not more fragile than X sperm when put in an acidic environment. He did have moderate success with his method, however. The problem is that his scientific reasoning and data collection processes were flawed. Since his theories about X and Y sperm were disproven, many researchers have sought to uncover a different method for sex-selection.

O +12 — A Flawed Method for Conceiving Girls

After Dr. Shettles' method didn't work for many parents, a group of researchers led by Dr. John France set out to investigate the accuracy of the Shettles method in New Zealand in 1984. This study

---

10   Penfold L. M., Holt, C., Holt, W. V., Welch, D. G., Cran, D. G., and Johnson, L. A. "Comparative motility of X and Y chromosome-bearing bovine sperm separated on the basis of DNA content by flow sorting." *Molecular Reproduction and Development* 1998; 50: 323-7.

11   Grant, V. J. "Entrenched misinformation about X and Y sperm." *BMJ* 332.7546 (2006): 916.

reported *opposite* results compared to those of Dr. Shettles. Out of 185 people, 52 live births resulted. The researchers eliminated 19 of those 52 births from the study for various reasons. The remaining 33 births were analyzed. They found that the only day during the menstrual cycle on which significantly more females than males were conceived was the day of ovulation and the day after. From these results, a new sex-selection method was born: "O+12" pronounced "oh plus twelve," referring to having sex 12 hours after ovulation in order to conceive a girl.[12]

The women in this study were instructed to track their LH surges, basal body temperatures (BBT) and cervical mucus in order to detect ovulation. Unfortunately, there was no relationship between the sex of the baby and timing intercourse relative to the day of the ovulation as detected by LH or BBT. The only relationship the researchers found was between the sex of the baby and the timing intercourse in relation to "peak cervical mucus secretions." The problem is, observing cervical mucus is a subjective and highly variable ovulation detection method.

A major flaw in this study is that the LH was only measured once daily using "first morning urine." I will explain the significance of this in the chapter, "Testing for Luteinizing Hormone", but for now, just know that testing only once a day results in unreliable LH surge detection.

The most critical flaw of the study was that the couples chosen for the study were not highly motivated to conceive a baby of a certain sex. Couples had an average of 2 children before they entered the study, with 6.5 boys for every 5 girls. Out of the 185 couples who entered the study, 85 couples dropped out, citing various reasons including: the couple no longer wanted to get pregnant, the study requirements were too hard, and the study was too stressful. Furthermore, out of the 52 births, a whopping 19 births were excluded from the study,

---

12   France, J. T., et al. "A prospective study of the preselction of the sex of offspring." *Fertility and Sterility* 41 (1984): 894-900.

because those parents failed to comply with the instructions, that is, even though they were instructed to have sex only once during the cycle, they had actually had sex multiple times. This resulted in the researchers' inability to pinpoint the specific act of intercourse that led to conception. To sum it up, 46% of the couples dropped out of the study right at the beginning, and of the remaining couples, 37% of them failed to follow the rules. Sounds like an unmotivated bunch of people. The reason this is such an important flaw in this study is that unmotivated subjects lead to inaccurate recording and reporting of their behavior, which can dramatically skew the data. For these reasons, this study is unreliable.

Despite the fact that the data was flawed, the O+12 method grew in popularity. It also stood as a reminder that the Shettles method couldn't possibly work, as these two methods clearly opposed each another. The O+12 method recommends trying for a girl after ovulation has occurred. The Shettles method recommends the opposite. They can't both be true.

Ions, and Diets, and Douches — Oh My!

Because of these two confusing methods and the lack of any developments in the area of natural sex-selection, many websites, blogs and forums began to focus on the one thing women love to control — diet. The problem is, most of us are unsuccessful when it comes to diets. The body wants what it wants, especially when you are trying to get it ready for pregnancy.

One sex-selection diet theory is based on the minerals you get from the foods you eat. This theory was developed based on a study done by Annet Noorlander in 2010 in Holland.[13] Women

---

13   Noorlander, A. M., Geraedts, J. P., and Melissen, J. B. "Female gender pre-selection by maternal diet in combination with timing of sexual intercourse – a prospective study." *Reproductive BioMedicine Online* 21.6 (2010): 794-802.

who wanted to conceive a girl were instructed to have a diet high in calcium and magnesium and low in salt and potassium. 32 women completed the study and 81% of them gave birth to a girl. However, these successes were not the result of the diet alone. The researchers had also instructed the women to implement the Shettles method of having sex frequently up until 2-3 days before ovulation, and using an LH test to determine ovulation. Hmm, sounds like the timing may have been an essential part of this "diet" method.

Another sex-selection diet theory is based on ions, aka the acidity or alkalinity of the foods that you eat. The theory is that if you eat more acidic foods, your body will become more acidic. Your acidified cervical mucus will kill all the weak boy sperm, leaving only the female sperm to fertilize the egg. Conversely, if you eat more alkaline foods, your body will become more alkaline, which favors the boy and girl sperm equally, making it a race to the egg and the fastest sperm wins... wait, isn't that just more of the Shettles method?

An additional theory behind this diet is that eating alkaline foods will cause your egg to have a negative charge, which will attract positively charged Y sperm, whereas eating acidic foods will cause your egg to have a positive charge, which will attract the negatively charged X sperm. This "egg polarity" theory has never been proven, and frankly, it doesn't make any sense. If sperm had different electrical charges, this would be relatively simple to detect in a laboratory setting, and scientists would have already exploited this difference in order to accurately sort sperm for artificial insemination.

On to the douches... where do I even start? This idea also relies on the acidic/alkaline theory that an acidic environment would kill the boy sperm, resulting in a female baby, and an alkaline environment would allow both sperm types to live, but the boy sperm would get to the egg first. To conceive a girl using this method, you would simply insert a lime-soaked tampon or a syringe full of lemon juice or something else acidic into your vagina before and after you have sex. This would supposedly acidify your vagina, kill the boy sperm, and allow only the girl sperm through. Conversely, to conceive a boy, you would just rinse your vagina with a baking soda douche to alkalize the environment, and the faster boy sperm will win. WHAT?? Sure, right before you go to make love to your man, you have to insert some burning acid or fizzing baking soda first. These sound like the absolute grossest, most uncomfortable, most dangerous things you could put into your vagina, right before it is about to become a pathway to conceiving another human life. Not to mention, humans have been able to successfully conceive both boys and girls without ever using a douche. And again, this acidic/alkaline idea came from Dr. Shettles.

The beauty of these websites focusing on ions, diets, and douches is that if the desired sex is not achieved, there's an easy rationalization. A woman may think to herself, "I guess I didn't follow the diet closely enough," or "I should have eaten more cranberries," or "Maybe I should have purchased the lime douche instead of the vinegar-lemon concoction." These methods are imprecise and have never been proven to work. Anecdotally, women post on message boards that eating a bunch of bananas worked, or having sex during a full moon worked, or doing cartwheels or jumping jacks or something else unscientific worked. Remember, the natural rate of boys and girls is basically 50/50, so of course some of these things appear to "work" and desperate people are willing to try anything. However, as a scientist myself, I prefer to rely on controlled trials and scientific evidence.

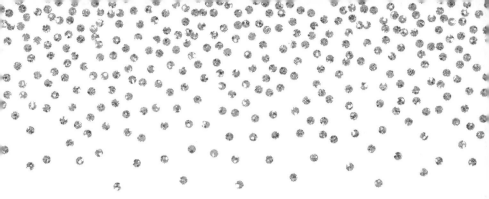

The Scientific Proof Behind
The Babydust Method

Timing, frequency, and LH charting are the essential components of *The Babydust Method.* I will now explain in detail the scientific proof behind *The Babydust Method,* and how you can use it to naturally and accurately choose the sex of your baby.

Timing is Everything

Timing is the cornerstone of *The Babydust Method.* The latest research indicates that the timing of sex in relation to ovulation is the most reliable method of sex selection. Several animal studies have shown that conception close to the time of ovulation produces significantly more males, whereas conception in the days before ovulation produces significantly more females. These studies have been done in cows, sheep, golden hamsters, and white-tailed deer.[14][15][16] I am highlighting the following studies below, as they have utilized the most rigorous study designs, methods, and data analyses.

Researchers studied how the timing of the insemination of female cows affected the sex of their calves.[17] When the cows began exhibiting the standard behavioral signs that indicated ovulation was approaching, researchers inseminated the cows at various time points: 12-22 hours before ovulation, 0-12 hours before ovulation, and right on ovulation. 73% of the cows inseminated in the 12-22 hours before ovulation gave birth to girls. Roughly the same amount of boys and girls resulted from the group of cows inseminated in the 0-12 hours before ovulation. 72% of the cows inseminated right on ovulation gave birth to boys. Keep in mind that the researchers were able to achieve these results by relying only on the cows' behavioral signs that ovulation was approaching. This is not a precise method of measuring ovulation, but it is pretty close. This study clearly proves the timing of intercourse in relation to ovulation influences the sex of the baby.

Another group of researchers did a similar study in cows, but in this study, the researchers used a vaginal probe to look at changes in the conductivity of the cervical mucus.[18] This is much more accurate

14   Gutiérrez-Adán, A., Pérez-Garnelo, S., Granados, J., Garde, J.j., Pérez-Guzmán, M., Pintado, B., and De La Fuente, J. "Relationship between sex ratio and time of insemination according to both time of ovulation and maturational state of oocyte." *Theriogenology* 51.1 (1999): 397.

15   Huck, U., William, J. S., and Lisk, R. D. "Litter sex ratios in the golden hamster vary with time of mating and litter size and are not binomially distributed." *Behavioral Ecology and Sociobiology* 26.2 (1990).

16   Verme, L. J., and Ozoga, J. J. "Sex ratio of white-tailed deer and the estrus cycle." *The Journal of Wildlife Management* 45.3 (1981): 710.

17   Martinez, F., Kaabi, M., Martinez-Pastor, F., Alvarez, M., Anel, E., Boixo, J. C., De Paz, P., and Anel, L. "Effect of the interval between estrus onset and artificial insemination on sex ratio and fertility in cattle: a field study." *Theriogenology* 62.7 (2004): 1264-270.

18   Wehner, G. R., Wood, C., Tague, A., Barker, D., and Hubert, H. "Efficiency of the OVATEC unit for estrus detection and calf sex control in beef cows." *Animal Reproduction Science* 46.1-2 (1997): 27-34.

than merely observing behavioral signs that indicate ovulation is approaching.[19] The researchers inseminated a group of cows when cervical mucus conductivity indicated ovulation was 20 hours away, and they inseminated another group of cows between the 8 hours before ovulation and the 8 hours after ovulation. Cows that were part of the group that was inseminated far in advance of ovulation went on to deliver 93% female calves. Cows that were inseminated right around ovulation delivered 92% male calves. This study proves that insemination before ovulation produces significantly more females, and insemination on ovulation produces significantly more males.

In this study, the researchers obviously didn't force the cows to eat bananas every day, or use different sexual positions, or change the degree of penetration, or insert lime-soaked tampons. It should be clear now that no diets, douches or special sexual maneuvers are necessary or effective in sex-selection.

Similar results were found in several other animal studies. The timing method works for cows, hamsters, deer, and sheep. How well does it work in humans? Glad you asked ;)

A study was done in 2011 by Dr. Leonie McSweeney with 99 couples who were interested in sex selection.[20] 81 couples wanted boys, and 18 wanted girls. The researchers noted that all the couples in the study were "highly motivated." Couples were selected based on who turned in their forms the fastest. Incidentally, of the 81 couples who wanted to conceive a male child, 24 couples did not yet have a son, and had between 2 and 8 daughters already. This was an extremely motivated group of individuals, don't you agree?

---

19   Straub, E. A., Edgerton, L. A., and Heershe, G. "Changes in electrical resistance of the vagina during estrus in heifers." *Preliminary report to Animark*, University of Kentucky-Lexington, 1984.

20   McSweeney, L. "Successful sex pre-selection using natural family planning." *African Journal of Reproductive Health* 15.1 (2011): 79-84.

All couples were instructed to wait 4 months after discontinuing breastfeeding, oral contraception, and IUDs, before attempting to conceive. This was to ensure hormone levels were back to normal. Women were instructed to check their cervical mucus secretions multiple times every day. Right after a woman's period, the cervical mucus present is sticky and creamy. After a few days, it starts to change to a more watery and slippery consistency. Cervical mucus remains watery and slippery until around ovulation when it changes back to sticky, creamy, or even non-existent. The last day of the slippery, watery consistency was to be noted as the "peak day." Women were instructed to record their mucus readings from the end of their period until a few days after their peak day. Women were told to chart these readings for 3 cycles before attempting conception.

Couples who wanted a girl were instructed to abstain from sexual intercourse from the start of their period, and then have sex once on the first day they noticed their secretions were no longer dry and sticky, but had turned wet and slippery. After having sex on this one day, couples were told to abstain until the 4th day after the peak day, when the woman is no longer fertile. If this method did not result in conception, women were told to move the day of intercourse closer and closer to the peak day in subsequent cycles. This stepwise method resulted in 16 females born out of the 18 couples attempting to have a female, or 88.9%.

Couples who wanted a boy were instructed to abstain from sexual intercourse from the start of the woman's period until ovulation was detected using cervical mucus patterns. For their first conception attempt, they were instructed to only have sex once, on the second day after the peak day. Since this is unlikely to result in conception (in fact, it resulted in only 4 babies — all male) couples who did not conceive during that cycle were instructed to have sex on the first day after the peak day, and again the day after that. After trying this timing method for 4 cycles, the remaining couples who had not yet conceived were instructed to have sex on the peak day itself, as well as the next day. This stepwise method of having sex closer and closer to ovulation on 2 consecutive days resulted in 78 males out of 81, or 96.3%. Again, no diets, douches, or sexual maneuvers were necessary.

Dr. McSweeney concluded that having sex once, as many days as possible before ovulation will result in a girl. Having sex twice, (once a day, on consecutive days) as close as possible to ovulation will result in a boy. This timing and frequency method was 94.9% effective overall.

But wait, this is basically the same timing as Dr. Shettles' method. Wasn't that method disproven? Yes, the *science* behind Dr. Shettles' timing method was wrong. X and Y sperm swim at the same speed, and Y sperm are neither more fragile nor more susceptible to acidic secretions than X sperm. So how does Dr. Shettles' timing method still produce successful results?

It has been suggested that the reason the timing of intercourse influences the sex of the baby so strongly is due to the difference between X and Y sperm capacitation.[21][22][23][24][25] That is, X and Y sperm capacitate at different points in time. Y sperm capacitate first and become able to fertilize the egg first, and then deteriorate. X sperm begin to capacitate later and become able to fertilize the egg later, and then deteriorate as well. Having sex during ovulation results in a boy, because the Y sperm capacitate first, and only

21   Bedford, J. M. "Significance of the need for sperm capacitation before fertilization in eutherian mammals." *Biology of Reproduction* 28.1 (1983): 108-20.

22   Madrid-Bury, N., Fernández, R., Jiménez, A., Pérez-Garnelo, S., Moreira, P.N., Pintado, B., De La Fuente, J., and Gutiérrez-Adán, A. "Effect of ejaculate, bull, and a double swim-up sperm processing method on sperm sex ratio." *The Biology of Gametes and Early Embryos Zygote* 11.3 (2003): 229-35.

23   Wehner, G. R., Wood, C., Tague, A., Barker, D., and Hubert, H. "Efficiency of the OVATEC unit for estrus detection and calf sex control in beef cows." *Animal Reproduction Science* 46.1-2 (1997): 27-34.

24   Barczyk, A. "Sperm capacitation and primary sex ratio." *Medical Hypotheses* 56.6 (2001): 737-38.

25   Martinez, F., Kaabi, M., Martinez-Pastor, F., Alvarez, M., Anel, E., Boixo, J. C., De Paz, P., and Anel, L. "Effect of the interval between estrus onset and artificial insemination on sex ratio and fertility in cattle: a field study." *Theriogenology* 62.7 (2004): 1264-270.

the Y sperm will be ready to fertilize the egg when it is released. Conversely, having sex during the days leading up to ovulation results in a girl, because the Y sperm have already capacitated and died before the egg has even been released. The X sperm then begin to capacitate, and are ready to fertilize the egg when it is released days later, resulting in a female baby.

Remember, Dr. Shettles' timing and frequency produced a 75-80% success rate. Dr. McSweeney used the same timing as Dr. Shettles did, but used the opposite frequency, and was able to achieve a 95% success rate. Therefore, frequency is clearly a critical component of sex-selection.

Frequency is Essential

Dr. McSweeney stressed the importance of having sex on 2 consecutive days in order to conceive a male, because she had found in her prior research that couples having sex only once, and on the peak day, resulted in an equal number of males and females conceived, whereas couples having sex on the peak day *and* the next day significantly increased the chances of conceiving a male.[26] There is additional scientific proof that having sex on 2 consecutive days favors boys. Let's take a look at the science behind this assertion.

The fact that a single act of intercourse around the time of ovulation can lead to an *equal* number of males and females is the very reason why conflicting methods like the Shettles method and O+12 can coexist. Timing is not the only critical variable — frequency is just as important. The fact that multiple acts of intercourse around the time of ovulation favors boys, whereas a single act of intercourse around ovulation produces boys and girls equally is the main reason why Dr. Shettles' method was not as successful as it could have been. He recommended the opposite frequency: one act of intercourse on

---

26 McSweeney, L. "Successful sex pre-selection using natural family planning." *African Journal of Reproductive Health* 15.1 (2011): 79-84.

ovulation for a boy, and frequent intercourse in the days leading up to the cut-off day, 2-3 days before ovulation, for a girl. Postings on websites like, "I had sex one time right on ovulation and had a girl" or, "We were BDing like rabbits up until the cut-off day and we got a boy," are common complaints, because timing by itself does not influence the sex of the baby as accurately as when the correct timing *and* frequency are used.

But why would having sex two days in a row make any difference in sex-selection? In nature, the goal of intercourse is to have successful offspring, that is, offspring who will go on to mate and produce offspring of their own. The Trivers-Willard hypothesis in population biology asserts that parental dominance and condition influence the sex of the resultant offspring.[27] What does that mean?

Let's take the mating behavior of a population of horses for example. Let's say there are 5 female horses and 5 male horses. The 5 male horses would all be competing for the same 5 females, with 1 stronger male typically winning out over the 4 weaker males every time. This genetically strong male would likely mate with all 5 females multiple times, and would prevent the 4 weak males from mating at all. It would be advantageous for this strong male horse to conceive more sons than daughters, since his sons would inherit his dominant qualities and would most likely impregnate multiple females.

Out of the 4 remaining weak male horses, 1 lucky horse may get a rare opportunity to mate with a female. It would be advantageous for him to have his genetics pass on to a daughter, since she would have a fair chance of having a few babies of her own, regardless of whether she is weak or strong. The weak male horse would not want to produce a son, because his son would probably be weak as well, and would most likely have zero offspring of his own.

---

27   Trivers, R. L., and D. E. Willard. "Natural selection of parental ability to vary the sex ratio of offspring." *Science* 179.4068 (1973): 90-92.

How could the female's body know if she is mating with a strong or a weak male, and how could her body influence the sex of her offspring? The *frequency* of intercourse is the key. A strong male is likely to mate with her several times in succession, whereas a weak male may only get one chance to mate with her. More frequent mating is telling her body that she is copulating with a strong male whose genetics are best passed on to a son. Conversely, less frequent mating is telling her body that this male is weak. Therefore, having a daughter would produce the best chance for future offspring.

Studies have proven this hypothesis about frequency to be true in humans. More frequent intercourse favors Y sperm and less frequent intercourse favors X sperm.[28] This is because when semen from a prior act of intercourse is present, the resulting environment favors Y sperm. Specifically, if a woman has sex one day and her reproductive tract doesn't have enough time to flush out the debris and particles from her partner's semen before she has sex again, that first batch of semen will alter the fluids in her vagina to favor the Y sperm from a subsequent act of intercourse.

In fact, the presence of semen from a prior act of intercourse can so greatly favor a boy, that it may neutralize the effect of timing alone. For example, let's say you were trying for a girl, and you aimed to have sex multiple times between the end of your period and 2-3 days before ovulation, as recommended by Dr. Shettles. You would actually have a good chance of having a boy instead, because the multiple acts of intercourse could cancel out the girl-favoring effects of the cut-off method.[29] Conversely, if you were going for a boy, and you decided to wait until the time of ovulation to have your one act of intercourse for that cycle, as recommended by Dr. Shettles, you would still have a possibility of having a girl. This is because having

---

28   Martin, J. F. "Length of the Follicular Phase, Time of insemination, coital rate and the sex of offspring." *Human Reproduction* 12.3 (1997): 611-16.

29   Martin, J. F. "Hormonal and behavioral determinants of the secondary sex ratio." *Social Biology* 42.3-4 (1995): 226-38.

sex just once may not be enough by itself to ensure you conceive a boy. Having sex once a day, on two consecutive days helps to make the environment even more favorable to the Y sperm.

Another reason frequency of intercourse is essential in sex-selection is that it enhances the accuracy of the timing of sex in relation to ovulation when trying to conceive a boy. When the LH surge is detected, ovulation occurs somewhere between 24 and 48 hours later. Because of this variability, a little insurance is needed. For example, if a woman does in fact ovulate 24 hours after her LH surge, having sex on that day would result in a male conception. By the time she would be having sex again 24 hours later, she would have already conceived. If however, she ovulated closer to 48 hours after the LH surge, which is possible but not as likely, she would have covered all her bases by having sex both 24 hours and 48 hours after the LH surge. If she instead had sex only once, 24 hours after the LH surge was detected, when she was actually due to ovulate 48 hours after the LH surge, she would have inadvertently created a 1 day cut-off, which could result in a female baby.

LH is the Star of the Show

So, should we just follow the sex selection methods outlined in the McSweeney study? Not exactly. The main problem with her study is that she relied exclusively on cervical mucus to detect ovulation. Cervical mucus patterns are not always reliable, and patterns vary from woman to woman, and cycle to cycle. In Dr. McSweeney's study, an undisclosed number of couples were given the sex-selection instructions, and were told to send in their charts once they had conceived. This is how the 99 couples were chosen for the study. The problem with this study design is that it favored women whose cervical mucus secretions did in fact coincide with ovulation. These women were able to time intercourse accordingly *and* get pregnant.

Unfortunately, some women do not have reliable cervical mucus patterns that coincide with ovulation. A study found that using cervical mucus patterns to determine ovulation can be imprecise and inconsistent at times.[30] The issue here is that Dr. McSweeney only included the data from women who became pregnant. She did not use the data from those who had tried her method and failed to get pregnant at all. Women who were unable to detect cervical mucus consistently were also excluded from the study.

For example, women who were never able to detect cervical mucus, or who detected it inconsistently, would have had trouble timing intercourse in relation to the peak day. This could have caused the women either to have sex on the wrong day, or to fail to conceive in general. Either way, they wouldn't have been included in the study.

Another flaw in the study is that Dr. McSweeney was relying on cervical mucus patterns in order to *detect* ovulation. The problem here is that cervical mucus patterns do not *predict* ovulation, they only tell you once it has already occurred, in retrospect. This could easily lead to errors in timing.

Consider this example: let's say you always have your peak cervical mucus day, which is the last day you have wet secretions, on cd14, but in some cycles it is on cd13 and sometimes cd15. You're going for a boy, and you detect wet cervical mucus on cd14 as predicted, and you have sex with your partner that night, assuming your cervical mucus will be dry the next morning. But when you wake up, your cervical mucus is still wet and slippery, meaning you accidentally had sex on the day before the peak day, not the actual peak day. See how easy it is to get the timing wrong? A woman like this who had gotten pregnant but unfortunately used

---

30   Hilgers, T. W., Abraham, G. E., and Cavanaugh, D. "Natural family planning I. The peak symptom and estimated time of ovulation." Obstetrics and Gynecology 1978; 52:575-82.

the incorrect timing would not have been included in the study. The cervical mucus peak day is only known retrospectively, when looking back at a chart. It is easy to make a mistake, since cervical mucus does not *predict* ovulation.

Testing for the LH surge is the most reliable way to track ovulation, as it is the only hormone that *predicts* ovulation. This is because it is the actual hormone that triggers the release of the egg from your ovary. A natural family planning study showed that peak cervical mucus occurred during the 24 hours before ovulation only 48.3% of the time, whereas the peak in urinary LH occurred during the 24 hours before ovulation 100% of the time.[31] Therefore, testing your urine for LH is the most accurate and reliable predictor of ovulation.

The information in the next chapter will teach you how to accurately test and record the results of your LH test strips. This will pinpoint ovulation and your most fertile days for accurate sex-selection. Timing intercourse according to your predicted ovulation day, and having intercourse with the correct frequency will help you more accurately choose the sex of your baby.

---

31 Guida M., Tommaselli G. A., Palomba S., et al. "Efficacy of methods for determining ovulation in a natural family planning program." Fertility and Sterility 1999;72:900-4.

Summary of *The Babydust Method*

Timing is everything. Frequency is essential. LH is the star of the show.

- **Summary of timing:** Animal and human studies have proven that having sex in the days leading up to ovulation results in a girl, and having sex as close to ovulation as possible results in a boy.

- **Summary of frequency:** Laboratory experiments and human studies have shown that a *single* act of intercourse most often results in a girl, while having intercourse *twice* most often results in a boy.

- **Summary of LH tracking:** Precise ovulation *prediction* is required. Tracking your LH surge using test strips is the most accurate and reliable way to predict ovulation. Testing and charting methods are detailed in the following chapters.

Testing for Luteinizing Hormone

Luteinizing hormone is the most reliable predictor of ovulation, and studies show that for the majority of women, ovulation typically occurs around 24 hours after the onset of the LH surge, with a range of 12-48 hours.[32] In this chapter, the procedure for testing for LH will be explained in detail. The next chapter, "Charting," will teach you how to record this data, and how to draw patterns from observing your cycle.

Testing — Aka POAS: Pee On A Stick

You must test for LH at least twice per day. Once with your first morning urine (FMU) or urine that has been held for at least 3 hours, and once at the end of the day, also with urine that has

---

32   "Ovulation kits & fertility monitors." *American Pregnancy Association*. N.p., 23 Apr. 2012. Web. 14 Mar. 2016.

been held for 3 hours. If you're like me, holding your pee for 3 hours sounds like absolute torture. When I'm home with the kids, I swear I pee every 15 minutes. Try to hold for at least an hour, and limit your fluid intake in the hours before you test. The reason for this is that the tests rely on the concentration of LH in your urine. An extra glass of water or a cup of coffee will dilute your urine and negatively affect your test strip.

You'll need about 10-20 LH test strips for each cycle. *The Babydust Method* tests are available on Amazon, only in the US at the moment, but any test strips with great reviews will work just fine! Try to limit your intake of liquid on the evenings prior to all testing days, so that you don't have to wake up to pee in the middle of the night. You don't want to have to pee in a cup and do an LH test strip at 2AM. Of course, waking up in the middle of the night to pee will happen from time to time (especially when you're pregnant — so get used to it!). However, if there will be more than 3 hours between your middle of the night pee and the time your alarm clock goes off, then it's fine to wait until the morning to take the test. For example, if you wake up at 2AM to go pee, but you know you'll be getting up at 6AM and will go pee again at that time, it is fine to use the 6AM urine as your FMU for testing. On the other hand, if you get up to pee at 5AM and you know you'll only go back to sleep until 6AM, then pee in a cup at 5AM and place it on your bathroom counter. When you wake up at 6AM, you can do the LH test on the 5AM sample. The morning test is the most important because you've been holding your urine the longest.

The second test of the day should be done in the evening hours before you go to bed. Testing at least twice a day is critical, because if you only test once a day, you may detect and record your LH surge much later than it actually occurred, or even worse, you could miss your surge completely. This is possible, because some women have an LH surge that lasts less than 24 hours. For example, let's say you only test once a day at 7AM. You test negative, but your LH surge actually begins 3 hours later, at 10AM. You might surge all day and all night and then stop surging around 5 in the morning the next day. Your 7ᴬᴹ test that day will be too late to catch the surge. Or, let's say you are still surging at 7ᴬᴹ that day. Since you tested negative yesterday at 7ᴬᴹ, you will assume your 7ᴬᴹ test today is the *start* of your surge, when in actuality your surge began at 10ᴬᴹ yesterday. By testing at least twice a day, you are more likely to catch the surge as soon as it begins.

Using *The Babydust Method* LH tests is easy. Tear off the top of the wrapper, and hold the stick by the colored handle. Dip the stick in your cup of urine until the top of the urine touches the "max line" on the strip and slowly count to 3. Take the strip out and lay it across the top of the cup or on top of the wrapper. Make sure it stays flat and horizontal while you wait 5 minutes for the strip to process. As it is processing, you'll see a faint pinkish/reddish dye moving across the strip. After 5 minutes, the dye will have stuck to the strip in two places: the result line and the control line. The result line is the line closest to the part of the stick you dipped into your urine, and the control line is the line closest to the colored handle of the stick. The control line will always turn dark red or maroon, whereas the result line varies between faint pink and dark maroon, depending on how close you are to your LH surge. The control line is just there for you to compare your result line to, and to show you that the test worked properly.

LH TEST INSTRUCTIONS

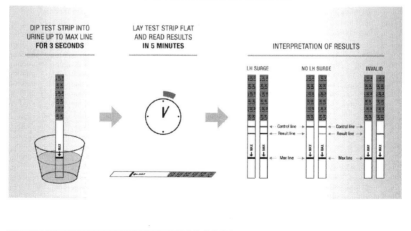

- **Faint:** The first few tests of your cycle will have a result line that is faint pink. Classify this result line in your calendar notes as "faint." This is your baseline level of LH when you are not yet surging. Continue testing twice per day.

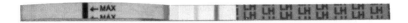

- **Medium:** If your result line is a medium pink or red color, meaning it is a little darker than your baseline "faint" reading, but is only about half as dark as the control line, call it "medium." This may occur 1-2 days before the surge, just hours before the surge, or you may never even see this medium color. You may just go straight from "faint" to "dark." If you do see this medium result line, it indicates your surge is approaching. Be diligent about testing at least twice per day. You want to catch the beginning of your surge, so more frequent testing at this point is beneficial.

- **Dark:** The definition of "dark" is very different from "medium." When you're looking at your result and control lines and the two lines are identical, or the result line is even darker than the control line, this indicates that your test is positive, and your LH is surging! You are not yet ovulating though, since ovulation takes place around 24 hours after the surge.

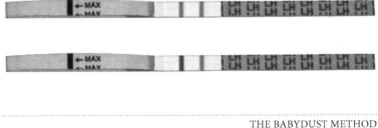

NOTE: To identify your positive, we're looking for your DARKEST test. Let's say you get a few medium tests, and then a test with equal lines. Don't assume this is your positive! Keep testing all the way through your surge until the test line goes back to faint. That way, you'll know you caught your absolute darkest test. For some women, the result line will get much darker than the control line, for others, a test with two equal lines is the darkest. Also, if you have a few tests that are all your darkest, meaning they're the darkest you get all cycle and they're all identical, indistinguishable from one another, you'd take the FIRST DARKEST test as your positive.

It's important to note that the length of your surge does not affect when the egg is actually released. Whether your surge lasts a few hours or a few days, always assume ovulation will occur 24 hours after your darkest test for the purposes of this method.

The tests are fully developed after about 5 minutes. Take photos of your tests at this point, because after 30 minutes, the tests will no longer be accurate. Using photos of your prior tests for comparison can help you notice patterns and chart more accurately.

Other Ovulation Tests and

the Importance of Frequent Testing

Digital ovulation tests from the drug store ovulation are not precise enough to use for sex-selection. You need to be able to see the subtle changes in the darkness of your result line in order to accurately predict ovulation for sex-selection.

For example, let's say you tested in the morning and got a negative result on your drug store test. If you had instead used test strips like *The Babydust Method* ovulation sticks, you could have seen the usually faint result line was more of a medium intensity that day. This is still a negative reading, but it indicates a changing level in LH, and that you're going to surge very soon. *The Babydust Method* tests are more precise, and can give you more advanced notice that your LH surge is approaching.

Another problem with using the drug store ovulation tests is that the instructions recommend testing just *once* a day. This could be partly because of the cost, but also because the tests are not meant to provide the precision that sex-selection requires. Testing only once a day could result in an almost 24 hour delay in detecting your surge, or you may miss detecting your surge completely. Remember the example explained earlier in this chapter? It's worth repeating: let's say you test at 7am and you get a negative result on your expensive test. You might have your LH surge just a few hours later at 10am, but you won't pick up that positive result until the next morning when you test again at 7am! The advantage of testing multiple times a day is that you catch your surge within hours of its onset. This is critical for sex-selection.

A Note on "Mittelschmerz"

Mittelschmerz, which is German for "middle pain," is felt during ovulation by 20% of women.[33] It is a sharp stabbing or throbbing sensation on either the left or the right side of your abdomen close to your hip bone, which is where your ovaries are located. You may think, "Well I can just feel ovulation happening, so I don't need to test for LH." This is an incorrect assumption. The exact cause of mittelschmerz is unknown, and while it could be the actual egg rupturing from the ovary, it could also be secondary causes of pain occurring long before or after the egg has already been released. Relying on this pain is not an accurate enough ovulation detection method.

---

33   "Mittelschmerz." *Mayo Clinic*. N.p., 30 May 2014. Web. 14 Mar. 2016.

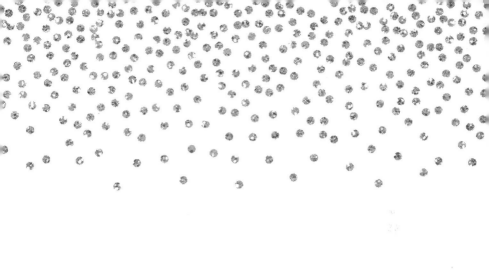

Charting

Let's start by tracking 3 practice cycles. If you have had a baby within the last 6 months, or if you have just stopped breastfeeding, chart 3 *extra* cycles (6 cycles total) before you begin your sex-selection attempt. I know that sounds like a long time to wait before you try to conceive, but your hormones are going through intense changes during the months following birth and weaning, and this could throw off your timing.

The calendar in the back of this book has space for you to record the date, the first day of your period, your LH testing results, and your BDing, or "baby dancing," aka having sex. Again, make sure you are not using birth control pills or an IUD for contraception, because these interfere with ovulation. During your practice cycles you are trying NOT to get pregnant. Therefore, you either need to use condoms or abstain from sexual intercourse. Your practice charting cycles are meant for you to gather data to use during your sex-selection cycle, which is when you're actually trying to get pregnant and choose the sex of your baby.

Charting Practice

Let's practice filling out a sample chart together. The following charts are based on a 28 day cycle. Let's say you just got your period on Friday the 4th. Write down, "Period," and, "cd1," (cycle day 1) on the 4th. Fill out the remaining cycle days, cd2-cd28 on the calendar.

MONTH 1   CYCLE DAYS FILLED IN

SUN	MON	TUE	WED	THU	FRI	SAT
		1	2	3	4 cd1-period	5 cd2
6 cd3	7 cd4	8 cd5	9 cd6	10 cd7	11 cd8	12 cd9
13 cd10	14 cd11	15 cd12	16 cd13	17 cd14	18 cd15	19 cd16
20 cd17	21 cd18	22 cd19	23 cd20	24 cd21	25 cd22	26 cd23
27 cd24	28 cd25	29 cd26	30 cd27	31 cd28		
NOTES:						

You will begin testing on cd5 with the LH test strips. Depending on the length of your cycle, you may need to continue to test until cd23 or even longer. You're just learning about the patterns of your cycle at this point. Test for LH *at least* twice a day. The more tests you take, the closer you'll get to detecting the absolute beginning of your surge. Fill in your test data every day from cd5 until you detect your LH surge.

Record your LH testing results in the morning and evening every day. Use "faint," "medium," or "dark" to indicate the shade of red of the result line (see previous chapter, "Testing for Luteinizing Hormone," for more detail). Let's say in this charting example, after recording several days of "faint" test results, your LH result line got a little darker than usual at 7ᴾᴹ on cd12. You determine it is only "medium" in tone, and is therefore not a positive result, but it does indicate your LH surge is likely approaching. Record this result as "medium" on your chart at 7ᴾᴹ on cd12. Remember, you may never get a medium test line, but if you *do*, it will occur right before you detect your LH surge.

MONTH 1   BEGAN TESTING, RECORDED RESULTS

SUN	MON	TUE	WED	THU	FRI	SAT
		1	2	3	4 cd1-period	5 cd2
6 cd3	7 cd4	8 cd5 begin testing LH 7ᴬᴹ faint 7ᴾᴹ faint	9 cd6 7ᴬᴹ faint 7ᴾᴹ faint	10 cd7 7ᴬᴹ faint 7ᴾᴹ faint	11 cd8 7ᴬᴹ faint 7ᴾᴹ faint	12 cd9 7ᴬᴹ faint 7ᴾᴹ faint
13 cd10 7ᴬᴹ faint 7ᴾᴹ faint	14 cd11 7ᴬᴹ faint 7ᴾᴹ faint	15 cd12 7ᴬᴹ faint 7ᴾᴹ medium	16 cd13	17 cd14	18 cd15	19 cd16
20 cd17	21 cd18	22 cd19	23 cd20	24 cd21	25 cd22	26 cd23
27 cd24	28 cd25	29 cd26	30 cd27	31 cd28		

NOTES:

Continuing with this example cycle, let's say you get your positive LH surge, that is, the result line is as dark as, or darker than the control line, at 7ᴬᴹ on cd13. You note this as "dark, LH surge." Since ovulation typically occurs 24 hours after the LH surge is detected, note "ovulation" on the calendar at 7ᴬᴹ on cd14. Since you have just detected your surge, you can stop testing for LH this cycle.

MONTH 1 — LH SURGE DETECTED, OVULATION NOTED

SUN	MON	TUE	WED	THU	FRI	SAT
		1	2	3	4 cd1-period	5 cd2
6 cd3	7 cd4	8 cd5 begin testing LH 7ᴬᴹ faint 7ᴾᴹ faint	9 cd6 7ᴬᴹ faint 7ᴾᴹ faint	10 cd7 7ᴬᴹ faint 7ᴾᴹ faint	11 cd8 7ᴬᴹ faint 7ᴾᴹ faint	12 cd9 7ᴬᴹ faint 7ᴾᴹ faint
13 cd10 7ᴬᴹ faint 7ᴾᴹ faint	14 cd11 7ᴬᴹ faint 7ᴾᴹ faint	15 cd12 7ᴬᴹ faint 7ᴾᴹ medium	16 cd13 7:00ᴬᴹ dark LH surge	17 cd14 7:00ᴬᴹ ovulation	18 cd15	19 cd16
20 cd17	21 cd18	22 cd19	23 cd20	24 cd21	25 cd22	26 cd23
27 cd24	28 cd25	29 cd26	30 cd27	31 cd28		

NOTES:

Now that you have your ovulation day determined, fill in the remaining days of the chart with "dpo," aka days past ovulation, with 1dpo being the day after ovulation. In this case, 1dpo is on cd15. The dpo days are used to determine which day to start testing for pregnancy. However, the first 3 cycles are just your practice charting cycles, and you will not be trying to get pregnant yet. You're just practicing filling out your calendar so you'll be ready for your sex-selection cycle.

MONTH 1   **DPO DAYS FILLED IN**

SUN	MON	TUE	WED	THU	FRI	SAT
		1	2	3	4 cd1-period	5 cd2
6 cd3	7 cd4	8 cd5 begin testing LH 7ᴬᴹ faint 7ᴾᴹ faint	9 cd6 7ᴬᴹ faint 7ᴾᴹ faint	10 cd7 7ᴬᴹ faint 7ᴾᴹ faint	11 cd8 7ᴬᴹ faint 7ᴾᴹ faint	12 cd9 7ᴬᴹ faint 7ᴾᴹ faint
13 cd10 7ᴬᴹ faint 7ᴾᴹ faint	14 cd11 7ᴬᴹ faint 7ᴾᴹ faint	15 cd12 7ᴬᴹ faint 7ᴾᴹ medium	16 cd13 7:00ᴬᴹ dark LH surge	17 cd14 7:00ᴬᴹ ovulation	18 cd15 1dpo	19 cd16 2dpo
20 cd17 3dpo	21 cd18 4dpo	22 cd19 5dpo	23 cd20 6dpo	24 cd21 7dpo	25 cd22 8dpo	26 cd23 9dpo
27 cd24 10dpo	28 cd25 11dpo	29 cd26 12dpo	30 cd27 13dpo	31 cd28 14dpo		

NOTES:

Record the cycle length and the LH surge day from this cycle in the space provided on the calendar. After 3 cycles of practice charting, you'll begin to notice your average cycle length and your average LH surge day. This is especially important when trying for a girl, because you will need to be able to predict when your LH surge will happen. It is also important to predict the day of your LH surge when trying for a boy, because you want to make sure you and your DP have cleared your calendars and are ready for BDing the day after your LH surge and the day after that. (Detailed example calendars are provided in the boy and girl chapters.)

CYCLE LENGTH: _____ DAYS
LH SURGE: CD_____

This practice cycle is now completely filled out. When you get your next period, go ahead and fill out the next month's cycle days, starting with "cd1" on the first day of your period. Make a note on cd5 to remind yourself to begin testing twice daily with your LH tests.

Recording BD "Activities"

Any time you have sex with your partner during your practice charting cycles, record it as "BD" (baby dance) on your calendar, so that you get used to tracking BDs. Remember, since you're not using an IUD or any kind of hormonal contraception, you MUST use a condom when you BD. Abstinence is of course preferable, as condoms are definitely not 100% effective in preventing pregnancy. It is much better to abstain from sexual intercourse entirely, until you are attempting to conceive during your sex-selection cycle. I know this is drastic, but it is the only way to ensure you don't get pregnant during your practice cycles.

Track your LH patterns for 3 cycles before you proceed with the boy or the girl method outlined in the following chapters. If after a few cycles, you haven't been able to detect ovulation using the LH test strips, bring your charting calendar in to your doctor for further analysis. Also, if you have noticed that the number of days between ovulation and the start of your next period is less than 10, bring your chart in to your doctor as well. You may have trouble getting pregnant with a short luteal phase, and there are drugs your doctor can prescribe to lengthen this part of your cycle.

It is important to read BOTH the boy and girl chapters no matter which one you are going for. If you are going for a girl, for example, it is critical to also read the boy chapter so you know what *not* to do.

THE BABYDUST METHOD

How to Conceive a BOY

Timing for a Boy

During your sex-selection cycle you will abstain from sex from day 1 of your period (cd1) until around the time of your positive LH test. This will typically be around 2 weeks. I know this may be too long for you and your DP to go without sex, but there are plenty of other things you can do to keep each other happy. Your DP can release on his own, or you can help him, and this can be done as frequently as your DP usually does. Just make sure he doesn't release any closer than 24 hours before your attempt, and don't let any sperm get near your vagina until your 2 sex-selection BDs. It's a small price to pay in order to have a precious baby boy in 9 months. It is absolutely critical that you abstain from sexual intercourse.

As I mentioned before, condoms are ok if you simply must have sex. However since this is your sex-selection cycle, even condoms can be detrimental, as it is unknown what role the chemicals on the outside of the condom may play in altering the environment in your vaginal tract. Also, since condoms are not 100% effective in preventing pregnancy, play it safe and abstain during these first two weeks of your sex-selection cycle.

Charting Example for a Boy

Let's say you got your period on Tuesday the 3rd. Note "cd1" and "period" on this day. Fill in the rest of your cycle days accordingly. You know from your 3 practice charting cycles that you usually get your positive LH test on cd13. So this month, make sure you and your DP will be available to BD around that day. Start testing on cd5, as you have been doing during your practice charting cycles.

Test for LH *at least* twice a day in order to detect the precise moment when your surge begins. Let's say, on the morning of cd13, you get your LH surge!! Now what? If you are surging on cd13 at 7ᴬᴹ, this means you'll ovulate on cd14 around 7ᴬᴹ. If you're going for a boy, you'll want to have your first BD as close to ovulation as possible, which would be around 7ᴬᴹ on cd14.

You don't need to BD *exactly* 24 hours after your positive LH test. If you tested positive at 7ᴬᴹ, you don't have to BD at 7ᴬᴹ the next day just to BD at the 24 hour mark exactly. Aim to have your first BD 24-30 hours after your positive test, getting as close as you can to 24 hours.

Frequency for a Boy

Ok, so you were able to have your first BD around 24 hours after your positive LH test? Perfection. Notate that on your chart. Your work isn't done yet, though. After your positive LH test, you need to BD at both 24 *and* 48 hours afterward. Remember, studies have shown that *two* acts of intercourse 24 hours apart will alter the uterine environment in favor of Y sperm. In the boy example chart, we said you tested positive on cd13 at 7ᴬᴹ, and you successfully BD'd around 24 hours after that, on cd14 at 7ᴬᴹ, which in this case is 24 hours after the surge. You'll want to BD *again* the following morning, cd15 at 7ᴬᴹ. Since you're going for a boy, you want to first BD as close to ovulation as possible, and BD a second time 24 hours after that. Remember, since you don't know when you ovulate exactly, BDing twice serves two purposes. One is to alter the environment to favor Y sperm, and the other is to ensure that you're BDing as close to ovulation as possible. Again, make sure your BDs are no closer than 24 hours apart, so that your DP's body has enough time to regenerate sperm to the count necessary to be able to even reach the egg. Notate your second successful BD on your chart.

MONTH 4 **GOING FOR A BOY (IDEAL)**

SUN	MON	TUE	WED	THU	FRI	SAT
1	2	3 cd1-period	4 cd2	5 cd3	6 cd4	7 cd5 begin testing LH 7ᴬᴹ faint 7ᴾᴹ faint
8 cd6 7ᴬᴹ faint 7ᴾᴹ faint	9 cd7 7ᴬᴹ faint 7ᴾᴹ faint	10 cd8 7ᴬᴹ faint 7ᴾᴹ faint	11 cd9 7ᴬᴹ faint 7ᴾᴹ faint	12 cd10 7ᴬᴹ faint 7ᴾᴹ faint	13 cd11 7ᴬᴹ faint 7ᴾᴹ faint	14 cd12 7ᴬᴹ faint 7ᴾᴹ medium
15 cd13 7ᴬᴹ dark LH surge	16 cd14 7ᴬᴹ BD#1 7ᴬᴹ ovulation	17 cd15 7ᴬᴹ BD#2	18 cd16	19 cd17	20 cd18	21 cd19
22 cd20	23 cd21	24 cd22	25 cd23	26 cd24	27 cd25	28 cd26
29 cd27	30 cd28					

NOTES:

For example, let's say you get your positive LH surge on cd13 at 7ᴬᴹ, and you do in fact ovulate the following morning on cd14 at 7ᴬᴹ right when you're BDing. That's great! If however, you actually ovulate closer to the 48 hour mark, just remember that the first BD will serve to make the environment more friendly to the Y sperm, and the second BD will ensure you get Y sperm up to the egg as close to the time of ovulation as possible. After your two well-timed BDs, you may continue to have unprotected sex as often as you like for the remainder of the cycle.

Remember, if you can't BD right at 24 hours after the LH strip first turned positive, aim to BD in the 24-30 hours after the positive LH test instead. If you're like me and have older kids in your house, BDing in the morning is next to impossible. Using the sample calendar as an example, if you can't BD in the morning on cd14, your next best bet would be before noon on cd14, and again 24 hours later on cd15.

MONTH 4   **GOING FOR A BOY (ALTERNATIVE)**

SUN	MON	TUE	WED	THU	FRI	SAT
1	2	3 cd1-period	4 cd2	5 cd3	6 cd4	7 cd5 begin testing LH 7ᴬᴹ faint 7ᴾᴹ faint
8 cd6 7ᴬᴹ faint 7ᴾᴹ faint	9 cd7 7ᴬᴹ faint 7ᴾᴹ faint	10 cd8 7ᴬᴹ faint 7ᴾᴹ faint	11 cd9 7ᴬᴹ faint 7ᴾᴹ faint	12 cd10 7ᴬᴹ faint 7ᴾᴹ faint	13 cd11 7ᴬᴹ faint 7ᴾᴹ faint	14 cd12 7ᴬᴹ faint 7ᴾᴹ medium
15 cd13 7ᴬᴹ dark LH surge	16 cd14 7ᴬᴹ ovulation 10ᴬᴹ BD#1	17 cd15 10ᴬᴹ BD#2	18 cd16	19 cd17	20 cd18	21 cd19
22 cd20	23 cd21	24 cd22	25 cd23	26 cd24	27 cd25	28 cd26
29 cd27	30 cd28					

NOTES:

After your two successfully timed BDs, fill in your dpo days for the rest of the chart. This is important, because you will use these dpos to decide which day to start taking your pregnancy tests. Since implantation occurs 6-10 days after ovulation, and the HCG level in your urine is detectable 3-4 days after that, the earliest you should test is 9dpo (more detailed information is in the chapter, "Am I Pregnant?!?! The 2WW and More POAS.")

SUN	MON	TUE	WED	THU	FRI	SAT
1	2	3 cd1-period	4 cd2	5 cd3	6 cd4	7 cd5 begin testing LH 7ᴬᴹ faint 7ᴾᴹ faint
8 cd6 7ᴬᴹ faint 7ᴾᴹ faint	9 cd7 7ᴬᴹ faint 7ᴾᴹ faint	10 cd8 7ᴬᴹ faint 7ᴾᴹ faint	11 cd9 7ᴬᴹ faint 7ᴾᴹ faint	12 cd10 7ᴬᴹ faint 7ᴾᴹ faint	13 cd11 7ᴬᴹ faint 7ᴾᴹ faint	14 cd12 7ᴬᴹ faint 7ᴾᴹ medium
15 cd13 7ᴬᴹ dark LH surge	16 cd14 7ᴬᴹ ovulation 10ᴬᴹ BD#1	17 cd15 10ᴬᴹ BD#2 1dpo	18 cd16 2dpo	19 cd17 3dpo	20 cd18 4dpo	21 cd19 5dpo
22 cd20 6dpo	23 cd21 7dpo	24 cd22 8dpo	25 cd23 begin testing HCG 9dpo	26 cd24 10dpo	27 cd25 11dpo	28 cd26 12dpo
29 cd27 13dpo	30 cd28 14dpo					

NOTES:

If you have not become pregnant after 2-4 cycles, try BDing closer and closer to the time you get your positive LH test. If you've already tried BDing at 24 and 48 hours after your surge, instead try 12 and 36 hours for 2-4 cycles. If that doesn't work, try immediately after the LH surge and 24 hours after that. Though rare, it is possible that you are someone who ovulates immediately after your surge is detected, and waiting until 24 hours after your surge for your first BD may be too late.

This is where the importance of testing *at least* twice a day comes in. The more tests you take, the closer you'll get to detecting the absolute beginning of your surge. If you instead test just once a day, you may catch your surge while it's already in progress. Waiting 24 hours from the *middle* of your LH surge to have your first BD may result in not getting pregnant at all. Be diligent, be scientific, and take control of your cycle.

There is no limit to the number of times you can test in a day. However, don't test so often that you become anxious. Anxiety about tracking your surge can cause it to be delayed. Your mind, diet, activity level, and sleeping habits can all negatively affect your cycle, primarily by delaying your LH surge and therefore delaying ovulation. Try to relax and let your body do its thing.

Helpful Hints

After BDing, don't get up right away. Stay horizontal, or better yet, prop up your hips with a pillow so your uterus is tilted. Don't get up for 10-30 minutes. Though sperm are excellent swimmers, you can help them out by making gravity less of a factor.

Please do not use Pre-Seed or any other lubricants. Anything you do to alter the natural environment in your vagina could affect your sex-selection attempt.

The average fertile couple only has a 25% chance of conceiving during any given cycle,[34] so don't get discouraged if it takes a few cycles to get pregnant. If you find yourselves trying to conceive for over a year, and you've already tried BDing right on the LH surge, then skip to the chapter, "General fertility: tips for getting pregnant with a girl OR a boy" and bring your charts to your doctor for review.

Boy Summary

After you get a dark result line on your LH test, which indicates you are surging, BD first around 24 hours and again around 48 hours after your positive test. Your goal is to BD *twice*, as close to ovulation as possible.

---

34   Imler, P., and Wilbanks, D. "The essential guide to getting pregnant." *American Pregnancy*, n.d. Web. 17 Mar. 2016.

How to Conceive a GIRL

Timing for a Girl

During your sex-selection cycle, you will abstain from sex from day 1 of your period (cd1) until you are 2-3 days before your predicted ovulation day. This will typically be around 10-20 days. I know this may be too long for you and your DP to go without sex, but there are plenty of other things you can do to keep each other happy. Your DP can release on his own, or you can help him, and this can be done as frequently as your DP usually does. Just make sure he doesn't release any closer than 24 hours before your attempt, and don't let any sperm get near your vagina until your BD attempt. It's a small price to pay in order to have a precious baby girl in 9 months. It is absolutely critical that you abstain from sexual intercourse.

As I mentioned before, condoms are ok if you simply must have sex. However since this is your sex-selection cycle, even condoms can be detrimental, as it is unknown what role the chemicals on the outside of the condom may play in altering the environment in your vaginal tract. Also, since condoms are not 100% effective in preventing pregnancy, play it safe and abstain during these first 10 days of your sex-selection cycle.

Charting Example for a Girl

Let's say you got your period on Tuesday the 3rd. Note "cd1" and "period" on this day. Fill in the rest of your cycle days accordingly. You know from your 3 practice charting cycles that you usually get your positive LH surge on cd13, so make sure you and your DP will be available to BD a few days before cd13.

In order to conceive a girl, you must start by BDing once, 2-3 days before your suspected ovulation. Notice I said *ovulation* not LH surge. Remember ovulation occurs around 24 hours *after* your positive LH test. So if you're supposed to BD 3 days before ovulation, then this really means you should BD 2 days before your predicted LH surge. This can be tricky, since the LH surge doesn't always happen on the same cycle day every month. For example, let's say during your 3 practice cycles, you got your LH surge on days 12, 14, and 13. Take your average LH surge day, which would be cd13 and subtract 2, which would be cd11. You would BD on cd11 to achieve a 3 day cut-off. Your predicted LH surge would be on cd13, your predicted ovulation would be on cd14, and you would be BDing on cd11, which would be 3 days away from cd14. Perfection :)

When calculating the day for your *one* BD, aka your cut-off day, half days are important. Let's say you always get your positive LH surge in the morning on cd13. Then you would count backwards 2 days to cd11 *in the morning*. So, you and your DP should BD on cd11 in the morning hours. Make sure you and your DP will be available then, and adjust your plans accordingly.

SUN	MON	TUE	WED	THU	FRI	SAT
1	2	3 cd1-period	4 cd2	5 cd3	6 cd4	7 cd5 begin testing LH 7ᴬᴹ faint 7ᴾᴹ faint
8 cd6 7ᴬᴹ faint 7ᴾᴹ faint	9 cd7 7ᴬᴹ faint 7ᴾᴹ faint	10 cd8 7ᴬᴹ faint 7ᴾᴹ faint	11 cd9 7ᴬᴹ faint 7ᴾᴹ faint	12 cd10 7ᴬᴹ faint 7ᴾᴹ faint	13 cd11 7ᴬᴹ faint 8ᴬᴹ BD #1 (the only BD)	14 cd12
15 cd13 (predicted LH surge: 7ᴬᴹ)	16 cd14 (predicted ovulation: 7ᴬᴹ)	17 cd15	18 cd16	19 cd17	20 cd18	21 cd19
22 cd20	23 cd21	24 cd22	25 cd23	26 cd24	27 cd25	28 cd26
29 cd27	30 cd28					

NOTES:

Now, if you're like me and have older kids in your house, BDing in the morning is next to impossible. If you cannot have sex in the morning for whatever reason, you could have sex in the evening on cd11, and still achieve a 2.5 day cut-off. This would still be perfection :)

SUN	MON	TUE	WED	THU	FRI	SAT
1	2	3 cd1-period	4 cd2	5 cd3	6 cd4	7 cd5 begin testing LH 7ᴬᴹ faint 7ᴾᴹ faint
8 cd6 7ᴬᴹ faint 7ᴾᴹ faint	9 cd7 7ᴬᴹ faint 7ᴾᴹ faint	10 cd8 7ᴬᴹ faint 7ᴾᴹ faint	11 cd9 7ᴬᴹ faint 7ᴾᴹ faint	12 cd10 7ᴬᴹ faint 7ᴾᴹ faint	13 cd11 7ᴬᴹ faint, 7ᴾᴹ faint 9ᴾᴹ BD #1 (the only BD)	14 cd12
15 cd13 (predicted LH surge: 7ᴬᴹ)	16 cd14 (predicted ovulation: 7ᴬᴹ)	17 cd15	18 cd16	19 cd17	20 c d18	21 cd19
22 cd20	23 cd21	24 cd22	25 cd23	26 cd24	27 cd25	28 cd26
29 cd27	30 cd28					

NOTES:

To sum it up, aim to BD 3 days before ovulation. If you cannot BD at exactly 3 days before your predicted ovulation, aim to BD sometime during the next 24 hours. This would still be in the girl range, since you would be BDing 2-3 days before ovulation.

If you have not become pregnant after 2-4 cycles using the 2.5-3 day cut-off, then try a 2-2.5 day cut-off for 2-4 cycles. If that doesn't result in pregnancy, try a 1.5-2 day cut-off. After that, try a 1 day cut off, which would mean BDing right on your LH surge. Though it is less common, it is possible that you are someone who ovulates closer to 48 hours after the surge is detected, and BDing a day or two before the surge is simply too far in advance of ovulation to get pregnant.

Now, it's possible that during your sex-selection cycle, you BD on the night of cd11 and then unexpectedly, on the morning of cd12 you get your positive LH surge, instead of on cd13 like you predicted. Don't worry! Remember, you ovulate 24 to 48 hours after the LH surge, so if you BD on cd11, test positive on cd12, and ovulate on cd13 or even cd14, you're still achieving a 2-3 day cut-off! Also, many women get several days of "faint" result lines before they get a "medium" result line. A "medium" result line indicates the LH surge is approaching, which can help you predict your LH surge far in advance. If you have irregular cycles, and calculating your average surge day is too difficult, mediums can indicate your surge is near.

When trying for a girl, it is critical that you test *at least* twice a day during your practice charting cycles. The more tests you take, the closer you'll get to detecting the absolute beginning of your surge. If you instead test just once a day during your practice cycles, you could catch your surge while it's already in progress, which would result in you recording your LH surge a day later than it actually occurred. This could lead you to BD too close to ovulation during your sex-selection cycle. Be diligent, be scientific, and take control of your cycle.

There is no limit to the number of times you can test in a day. However, don't test so often that you become anxious. Anxiety about tracking your surge can cause it to be delayed. Your mind, diet, activity level, and sleeping habits can all negatively affect your cycle, primarily by delaying your LH surge and therefore delaying ovulation. Try to relax and let your body do its thing.

Frequency for a Girl

As a reminder, once you determine your cut-off day based on your practice cycles, have sex *one* time and only on that day. After your one well-timed BD, do not have sex again until 7 days after the day you detected your LH surge. If abstinence is impossible, you may use condoms. However as I mentioned before, this may alter the environment in your vaginal tract, so abstinence is always better. On the calendar below, "resume BD ok" was noted on cd20, since that is 7 days after the LH surge was detected.

After your *one* successfully timed BD, and after you detect your LH surge, fill in your dpo days for the rest of the chart. This is important, because you will use these dpos to decide which day to start taking your pregnancy tests. Since implantation occurs 6-10 days after ovulation, and the HCG level in your urine is detectable 3-4 days after that, the earliest you should test is 9dpo (more detailed information is in the chapter, "Am I Pregnant?!?! The 2WW and More POAS.")

MONTH 4   CONTINUED TESTING, FILLED IN DPO DAYS, RESUMED BD

SUN	MON	TUE	WED	THU	FRI	SAT
1	2	3 cd1-period	4 cd2	5 cd3	6 cd4	7 cd5 begin testing LH 7ᴬᴹ faint 7ᴾᴹ faint
8 cd6 7ᴬᴹ faint 7ᴾᴹ faint	9 cd7 7ᴬᴹ faint 7ᴾᴹ faint	10 cd8 7ᴬᴹ faint 7ᴾᴹ faint	11 cd9 7ᴬᴹ faint 7ᴾᴹ faint	12 cd10 7ᴬᴹ faint 7ᴾᴹ faint	13 cd11 7ᴬᴹ faint 8ᴬᴹ BD #1 (the only BD)	14 cd12 7ᴬᴹ medium
15 cd13 7ᴬᴹ dark LH surge	16 cd14 7ᴬᴹ ovulation	17 cd15 1dpo	18 cd16 2dpo	19 cd17 3dpo	20 cd18 4dpo	21 cd19 5dpo
22 cd20 resume BD ok (7 days after LH) 6dpo	23 cd21 7dpo	24 cd22 8dpo	25 cd23 begin testing HCG 9dpo	26 cd24 10dpo	27 cd25 11dpo	28 cd26 12dpo
29 cd27 13dpo	30 cd28 14dpo					

NOTES:

Helpful Hints

After BDing, don't get up right away. Stay horizontal, or better yet, prop up your hips with a pillow so your uterus is tilted. Don't get up for 10-30 minutes. Though sperm are excellent swimmers, you can help them out by making gravity less of a factor.

Please do not use Pre-Seed or any other lubricants. Anything you do to alter the natural environment in your vagina could affect your sex-selection attempt.

The average fertile couple only has a 25% chance of conceiving during any given cycle,[35] so don't get discouraged if it takes a few cycles to get pregnant. If you find yourselves trying to conceive for over a year, and you've already tried BDing right on the LH surge, then skip to the chapter, "General fertility: tips for getting pregnant with a girl OR a boy" and bring your charts to your doctor for review.

Girl Summary

Your goal is to BD *once*, 2-3 days before your predicted ovulation day, using your past charts to predict ovulation.

---

35   Imler, P., and Wilbanks, D. "The essential guide to getting pregnant." *American Pregnancy*, n.d. Web. 17 Mar. 2016.

THE BABYDUST METHOD

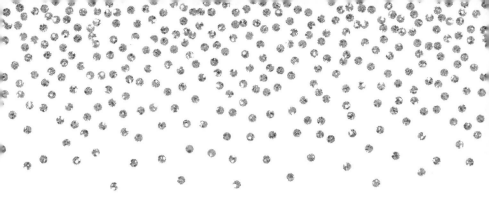

Am I Pregnant?!?!
The 2WW and More POAS

So, you timed your BD or BDs perfectly, now what? You have just entered the 2WW or "two week wait." This is the time after ovulation, but it's still too early to get a positive result on a pregnancy test. Yes, conception has possibly occurred, but your body doesn't know it yet. How is this possible? Let's take a look at the science of conception again.

Conception vs. Pregnancy

If the sperm and egg fuse together and form a zygote, then conception has occurred. The zygote starts dividing and becomes 2 cells, then 4, 8, and so on. Then, it buries itself into your uterine lining, where it will receive nourishment from your body. This is called *implantation*.

The blastocyst's journey from your fallopian tubes to your uterus takes 6-12 days, with implantation occurring most commonly on day 9.[36] As soon as the blastocyst implants, your body begins to produce human chorionic gonadotropin, aka HCG. This is the hormone that urine pregnancy tests rely on to determine pregnancy. At the moment of implantation, the level of HCG is not yet high enough in your urine to get an accurate result on a pregnancy test.

However, implantation itself may give you an early sign that you are pregnant. Some women notice pink or light brown spotting as a result of the blastocyst's interaction with the blood lining in your uterus during implantation. You may only see it on a tissue after you urinate, but don't worry if you don't see it at all. Be on the lookout for the spotting between 6dpo and 12dpo.

So, when can you start testing for HCG? (Use the example charts in the prior chapters for reference). The soonest that implantation can occur is 6dpo. Around 3-4 days after implantation, the level of HCG is high enough to be detected in your urine. So, the soonest you could test and expect a positive result, or BFP, aka "big fat positive," is 9dpo. Don't be discouraged if your test is negative, aka BFN, "big fat negative." You should continue to test daily, from 9dpo until you get your period. Of course people claim to have gotten BFPs as early as 5dpo. While this is extremely rare, and is probably due to an error in charting, do not begin testing until 9dpo. Even a POAS addict like myself needs to hold back.

To keep from going crazy during the 2WW, you can join, "The Babydust Method Group Forum," on Facebook! Many women are online, comparing early pregnancy symptoms and supporting each other during this tense time. Check out the posts on the Facebook group and connect with women who are going through this process and having the same feelings you are.

Once you get to 9dpo and can finally POAS, have your HCG strips ready. *The Babydust Method* tests are available on Amazon, only in the US at the moment, but any test strips with great reviews will work just fine!

36 "How soon after implantation do I get a positive pregnancy test?" *New Health Advisor*, N.p., n.d. Web. 14 Mar. 2016.

Just like the expensive drug store pregnancy tests, *The Babydust Method* strips test for an HCG level of 25 mIU/mL (milli-international units per milliliter). Just like LH tests, HCG tests rely on the concentration of the hormone in your urine, so use your FMU or urine that has been held for at least 3 hours. Try to limit your intake of liquid on the evenings before your morning tests. If you do wake up to pee, and it's less than 3 hours before getting up for the day, then just pee in a cup and place it on the bathroom counter. When you wake up later, you can do the HCG test on that urine.

Using the HCG tests is easy. Follow the same instructions you used for the LH tests. Tear off the top of the wrapper, and hold the stick by the colored handle. Dip the stick in your cup of urine until the top of the liquid hits the "max line" on the strip and slowly count to 3. Take the strip out and lay it across the top of the cup or on top of the wrapper. Make sure it stays flat and horizontal while you wait 5 minutes for the strip to process.

HCG TEST INSTRUCTIONS

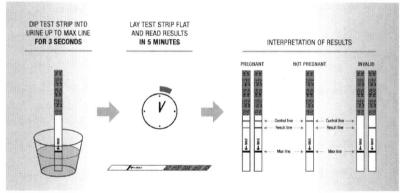

Just like the LH tests, the control line on the HCG tests will always turn dark red or maroon, whereas the result line could be non-existent, faint pink, medium red, or dark maroon. If there is no line at all, either you are not pregnant, or the concentration of HCG in your urine has not yet risen to a detectable level. Keep testing, you might test positive in a day or two. If there is *any* result line at all, even the faintest of pink lines, aka "a squinter", then you are PREGNANT!!! Go online and post a photo of your positive test — your BFP, or big fat positive!!

FAINT, MEDIUM, AS DARK, DARKER — ALL POSITIVE!!!

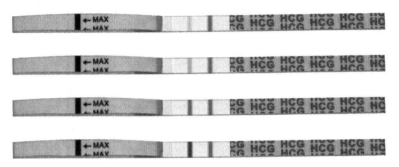

Just like the LH tests, the HCG tests depend on the concentration of the hormones in your urine. *Unlike* the LH tests however, the HCG tests do not require a dark result line to be positive. LH is present in your body at varying levels throughout your cycle, so you will likely get at least a faint result line on any given day. HCG on the other hand, is only produced if you are pregnant.

If you decide to continue to test in the days after getting your BFP, you will likely see the result line get darker and darker. But please, stop testing. You will be wasting tests, and you may even get confusing results. After a few days of getting dark lines, you may start to see the lines get lighter and lighter. This will cause you to absolutely freak out. This does not mean you are no longer pregnant. These tests are designed to read low levels of HCG. Let's say your first positive test detected a level of 30 mIU/mL in your urine. HCG levels double every few days, so by the end of the first week, you may have a level of 250, and by the next week you could have a level of 2,000. Because the test strips are meant to read low levels, they become overwhelmed by the extreme amount of HCG now present in your body. This causes the appearance of a scary negative reading on your test strip. Stop testing. You already know you're pregnant!!!

Ok, Now What?

Most OB/GYNs will not have you come into their office until you are 8 or 9 weeks pregnant, counting from the first day of your last menstrual period. It is critical that you continue to take your prenatal vitamins daily, and that you discontinue any unnecessary or harmful substances (eg. coffee, alcohol, cigarettes). This is the most vulnerable time of your baby's development, and it's all happening before you've even seen a doctor. Treat your body and your baby right.

THE BABYDUST METHOD

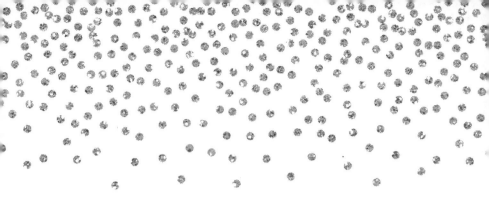

General Fertility:
Tips for Getting Pregnant
with a Boy OR a Girl

As I mentioned before, the average fertile couple only has a 25% chance of conceiving during any given cycle,[37] so don't get discouraged if it takes a few cycles to get pregnant. If you find yourselves trying to conceive for over a year, and you've already tried BDing as close as you can to the LH surge, for either the boy or the girl method, then you may decide it's time to focus on just getting pregnant.

Timing sex in order to get pregnant with either sex is much easier than timing sex specifically for a girl or a boy. Since you've already been charting your cycles, it should be easy to see when you're due to ovulate each month. Let's say you have a 28 day cycle,

---

37   Imler, P., and Wilbanks, D. "The essential guide to getting pregnant." *American Pregnancy,* n.d. Web. 17 Mar. 2016.

you usually get your positive LH test on cd13, and you assume you're ovulating on cd14. For maximum fertility, you should BD every other day or every third day from 5 days before your LH surge, until 3 days after your surge. In this example, you would BD frequently from cd8 until cd16, making sure to BD on cd13 and cd14, as those are your most fertile days. It's fine to BD throughout your cycle, just make sure you BD frequently during those 8 days.

Though it may sound counterintuitive, BDing *every* day may actually lower your DP's sperm count to the point of not being able to conceive. You need to give his body at least 24 hours in between BDs to build up the sperm count necessary to be able to reach the egg.

If you've been trying to conceive for over a year, make an appointment with your doctor and bring in your charts for review. Your doctor will analyze your overall health and give you specialized advice, and possibly a prescription for something to help you conceive.

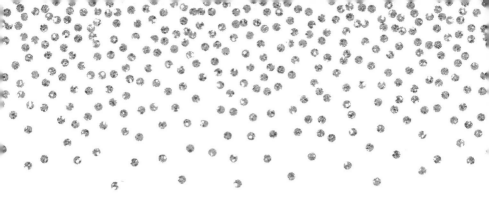

Fertility After Baby and Planning for Your Next Bundle of Joy

So, you successfully got pregnant and delivered your gorgeous little baby! Congratulations!! What's next for your family? If you're like me and didn't *love* being pregnant, you won't be thinking about getting pregnant again any time soon. After you've healed from giving birth and have settled into a routine with your little one, the time will come when you and your DP will resume having sex. Please, please, PLEASE have a method of birth control ready to go before you have sex. If you are not breastfeeding, get back on birth control pills, use condoms, or put in an IUD. If you *are* breastfeeding, there are lower dose birth control pills you can take that have been proven to have little or no effect on breast milk. And remember, birth control pills take a whole cycle before they are effective in preventing pregnancy, so use a backup method like condoms during your first cycle of getting back on birth control pills.

DO NOT use the charting methods from this book to attempt to *prevent* pregnancy by timing sex on your non-fertile days, aka the rhythm method. This is not a reliable method of preventing pregnancy. For example, if you have sex one day, assuming you're not fertile yet, and then the very next morning you get your positive LH surge, you could absolutely get pregnant. Sperm live up to 5-7 days inside you, so the sperm from that act of intercourse could be hanging around and waiting for your egg to be released, which could result in pregnancy. It is extremely important that you are using a reliable form of contraception, like birth control pills, condoms, or an IUD.

The reason I am so adamant about getting your contraception plan in place is that it is a MYTH that you cannot get pregnant if you are breastfeeding, and it is a MYTH that you cannot get pregnant if you have not yet gotten your period back. Once your period has come back, you were actually fertile when you ovulated approximately two weeks earlier. I cannot tell you how many friends have accidentally gotten pregnant because they assumed they were infertile, since they had not yet seen their periods resume. Having one child is a game-changer, a life-altering decision, so having two children in quick succession can be extremely difficult if you aren't ready. That's not to say families don't manage when they have an unexpected pregnancy — of course they can. Having a baby is a huge deal though, so it shouldn't be taken lightly. Take control of your cycle and your fertility.

I hope you'll be consulting *The Babydust Method* again (and again!) to select the sex of your next baby. In the meantime, check out, "The Babydust Method Group Forum," on Facebook. Post a question about the method, testing, or your personal situation. Post your success story, or even a photo of you and your new baby to the group page! It will help others see how effective the method was for you and encourage them to be just as diligent during their sex-selection cycle. You can connect with women who are just starting their sex-selection attempt, or who are awaiting their BFP in the 2WW. Bond with other women whose babies are in the same birth-month club as yours. Chat about breastfeeding, baby names, baby gear, and all things baby.

Babydust to all
XOXO,
Kathryn

Bibliography

- **Barczyk, A.** "Sperm capacitation and primary sex ratio." *Medical Hypotheses* 56.6 (2001): 737-38.

- **Bedford, J. M.** "Significance of the need for sperm capacitation before fertilization in eutherian mammals." *Biology of Reproduction* 28.1 (1983): 108-20.

- **Ben-Porath, Y., and Welch, F.** "Do sex preferences really matter?" *The Quarterly Journal of Economics* 90.2 (1976): 285.

- **France, J. T., et al.** "A prospective study of the preselction of the sex of offspring." *Fertility and Sterility* 41 (1984): 894-900.

- **Grant, V. J.** "Entrenched misinformation about X and Y sperm." *BMJ* 332.7546 (2006): 916.

- **Guida M., Tommaselli G. A., Palomba S., et al.** "Efficacy of methods for determining ovulation in a natural family planning program." *Fertility and Sterility* 1999;72:900-4.

- **Gutiérrez-Adán, A., Pérez-Garnelo, S., Granados, J., Garde, J.j., Pérez-Guzmán, M., Pintado, B., and De La Fuente, J.** "Relationship between sex ratio and time of insemination according to both time of ovulation and maturational state of oocyte." *Theriogenology* 51.1 (1999): 397.

- **Hilgers, T. W., Abraham, G. E., and Cavanaugh, D.** "Natural family planning I. The peak symptom and estimated time of ovulation." *Obstetrics and Gynecology* 1978; 52:575-82.

- **Hossain, A. M., Barik, S., and Kulkarni, P. M.** "Lack of significant morphological differences between human X and Y spermatozoa and their precursor cells (spermatids) exposed to different prehybridization treatments." *Journal of Andrology* 2001; 22: 119-23.

- "How soon after implantation do I get a positive pregnancy test?" *New Health Advisor*, N.p., n.d. Web. 14 Mar. 2016.

- **Huck, U., William, J. S., and Lisk, R. D.** "Litter sex ratios in the golden hamster vary with time of mating and litter size and are not binomially distributed." *Behavioral Ecology and Sociobiology* 26.2 (1990).

- **Imler, P., and Wilbanks, D.** "The essential guide to getting pregnant." *American Pregnancy*, n.d. Web. 17 Mar. 2016.

- **Johnson, L. A., Welch, G. R., Keyvanfar, K., Dorfmann, A., Fugger, E. F., and Schulman, J. D.** "Gender preselection in humans? Flow cytometric separation of X and Y spermatozoa for the prevention of X-linked diseases." *Human Reproduction* 1993, 8: 1733-1739.

- **Madrid-Bury, N., Fernández, R., Jiménez, A., Pérez-Garnelo, S., Moreira, P.N., Pintado, B., De La Fuente, J., and Gutiérrez-Adán, A.** "Effect of ejaculate, bull, and a double swim-up sperm processing method on sperm sex ratio." *The Biology of Gametes and Early Embryos Zygote* 11.3 (2003): 229-35.

- **Martin, J. F.** "Length of the Follicular Phase, Time of insemination, coital rate and the sex of offspring." *Human Reproduction* 12.3 (1997): 611-16.

- **Martin, J. F.** "Hormonal and behavioral determinants of the secondary sex ratio." *Social Biology* 42.3-4 (1995): 226-38.

- **Martinez, F., Kaabi, M., Martinez-Pastor, F., Alvarez, M., Anel, E., Boixo, J. C., De Paz, P., and Anel, L.** "Effect of the interval between estrus onset and artificial insemination on sex ratio and fertility in cattle: a field study." *Theriogenology* 62.7 (2004): 1264-270.

- "Mittelschmerz." *Mayo Clinic*. N.p., 30 May 2014. Web. 14 Mar. 2016.

- **McSweeney, L.** "Successful sex pre-selection using natural family planning." *African Journal of Reproductive Health* 15.1 (2011): 79-84.

- **Muehleis P. M.** "The effects of altering the pH of seminal fluid on the sex ratio of rabbit off- spring." *Fertility and Sterility* 1976, 27: 1438-45.

- **Noorlander, A. M., Geraedts, J. P., and Melissen, J. B.** "Female gender pre-selection by maternal diet in combination with timing of sexual intercourse – a prospective study." *Reproductive BioMedicine Online* 21.6 (2010): 794-802.

- "Ovulation kits & fertility monitors." *American Pregnancy Association.* N.p., 23 Apr. 2012. Web. 14 Mar. 2016.

- **Penfold L. M., Holt, C., Holt, W. V., Welch, D. G., Cran, D. G., and Johnson, L. A.** "Comparative motility of X and Y chromosome-bearing bovine sperm separated on the basis of DNA content by flow sorting." **Molecular Reproduction and Development** 1998; 50: 323-7.

- **Shettles, L. B., and Rorvik, D. M.** "How to choose the sex of your baby: the method best supported by scientific evidence." New York: Broadway, 2006.

- **Straub, E. A., Edgerton, L. A., and Heershe, G.** "Changes in electrical resistance of the vagina during estrus in heifers." *Preliminary report to Animark,* University of Kentucky-Lexington, 1984.

- **Trivers, R. L., and D. E. Willard.** "Natural selection of parental ability to vary the sex ratio of offspring." *Science* 179.4068 (1973): 90-92.

- **Verme, L. J., and Ozoga, J. J.** "Sex ratio of white-tailed deer and the estrus cycle." *The Journal of Wildlife Management* 45.3 (1981): 710.

- **Wehner, G. R., Wood, C., Tague, A., Barker, D., and Hubert, H.** "Efficiency of the OVATEC unit for estrus detection and calf sex control in beef cows." *Animal Reproduction Science* 46.1-2 (1997): 27-34.

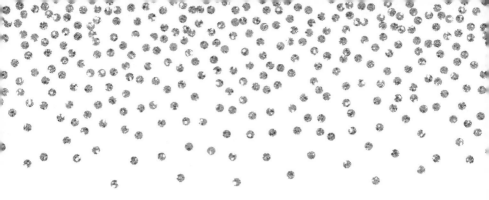

Blank Calendars
for Charting

MONTH _____

SUN	MON	TUE	WED	THU	FRI	SAT

CYCLE LENGTH: _____ DAYS

LH SURGE: CD _____

THE BABYDUST METHOD

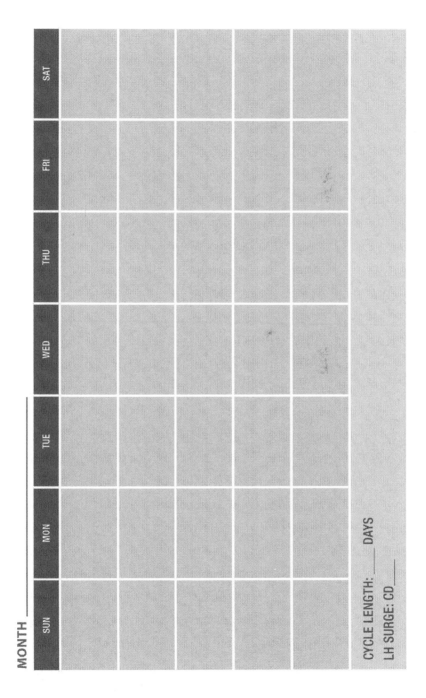

MONTH ___

SUN	MON	TUE	WED	THU	FRI	SAT

CYCLE LENGTH: ____ DAYS
LH SURGE: CD ____

SUN	MON	TUE	WED	THU	FRI	SAT

CYCLE LENGTH: _____ DAYS

LH SURGE: CD _____

MONTH _____

SUN	MON	TUE	WED	THU	FRI	SAT

CYCLE LENGTH: _____ DAYS

LH SURGE: CD _____

MONTH _____

SUN	MON	TUE	WED	THU	FRI	SAT

CYCLE LENGTH: _____ DAYS

LH SURGE: CD _____

THE BABYDUST METHOD

MONTH _____

SUN	MON	TUE	WED	THU	FRI	SAT

CYCLE LENGTH: _____ DAYS

LH SURGE: CD _____

MONTH _____

SUN	MON	TUE	WED	THU	FRI	SAT

CYCLE LENGTH: _____ DAYS

LH SURGE: CD _____

THE BABYDUST METHOD

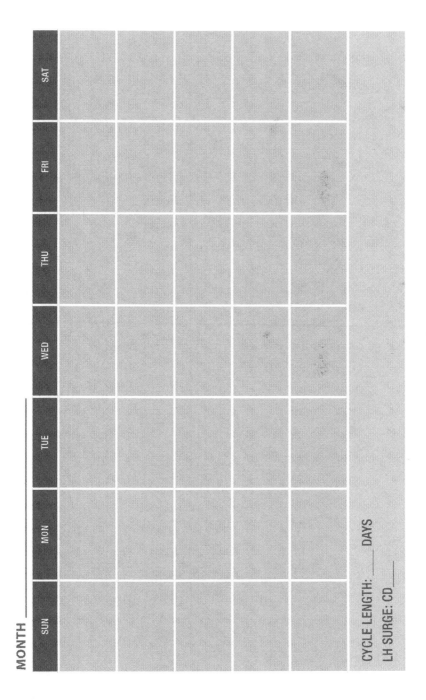

MONTH _____

SUN	MON	TUE	WED	THU	FRI	SAT

CYCLE LENGTH: _____ DAYS
LH SURGE: CD _____

MONTH _____

	SUN	MON	TUE	WED	THU	FRI	SAT

CYCLE LENGTH: _____ DAYS
LH SURGE: CD _____

THE BABYDUST METHOD

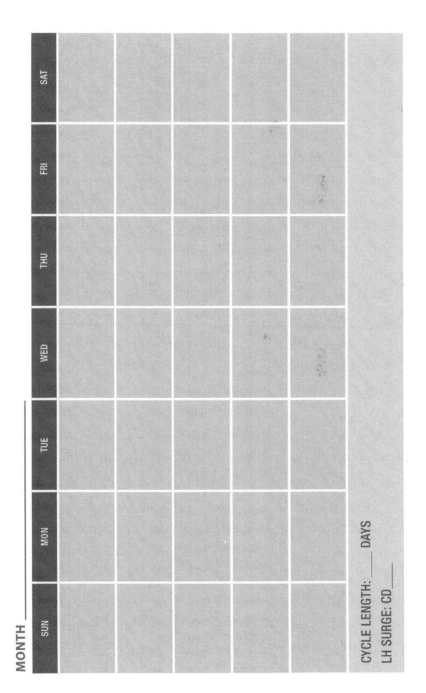

MONTH _____

SUN	MON	TUE	WED	THU	FRI	SAT

CYCLE LENGTH: _____ DAYS
LH SURGE: CD _____

MONTH _____

SUN	MON	TUE	WED	THU	FRI	SAT

CYCLE LENGTH: _____ DAYS

LH SURGE: CD _____

MONTH _____

SUN	MON	TUE	WED	THU	FRI	SAT

CYCLE LENGTH: _____ DAYS

LH SURGE: CD _____